Scottish Home and Health Department
Scottish Health Service Advisory Council

Prevention of Coronary Heart Disease in Scotland

Report of the Working Group on
Prevention and Health Promotion

Edinburgh   HMSO

ISBN 0 11 494111 4

Note by Scottish Home and Health Department

On 13 March 1990, Mr Michael Forsyth, Minister for Health at the Scottish Office, announced the Government's response to this report and to a review of health education in Scotland, carried out by management consultants. Mr Forsyth welcomed the capable work of the Working Group and acknowledged the significance of their findings. On the basis of the Group's conclusions and the recommendations from the more general review, the Minister announced *inter alia* that:

i.   a national policy statement would be prepared on health education with a positive orientation towards health promotion;

ii.   a new national health education organisation would be established with effect from 1 April 1991, separate from the Common Services Agency, and charged with implementing the national policy statement;

iii. the prevention of coronary heart disease would be one of the specific subjects which would be addressed in the national policy statement;

iv.   the details of the proposed individual approach recommended by the Working Group would be carefully examined and taken into account in the development of the Government's approach to coronary heart disease prevention.

Chairman's Foreword

In June 1988 the Scottish Health Service Planning Council decided to establish a series of Working Groups to examine how best to reduce morbidity within the population of Scotland. In view of the fact that coronary heart disease was known to be a major cause of premature death in Scotland the Planning Council decided to set up our group to assess the current position regarding coronary heart disease and specifically to 'review the issues relating to the prevention of coronary heart disease'.

The model which we recommend is based on a population approach providing a backdrop against which is would become easier for individuals to respond to specific advice contained in the individual strategy regarding the prevention of coronary heart disease. One of the exciting recommendations of our report must be that concerned with the establishment of a new body directly responsible for health promotion.

Having taken oral advice from a variety of sources and having received written evidence from several bodies, identified in the report, we decided to form two sub-groups to take forward the separate issues of the population approach and the individual strategy. Dr H J Dargie chaired the Individual Strategy Group while the Population Group was chaired by Dr W C Smith.

I am indebted to the whole group for its stimulating contributions and particularly grateful to Dr Dargie and Dr Smith not only for their work with the sub-groups but also for their invaluable help and advice throughout the entire exercise. I wish also to place on record my thanks to the Assessors for their wisdom and help. I am extremely indebted to Mrs F M Cruickshanks, Scottish Health Service Advisory Council Secretariat for her ever helpful efficiency.

W Keith Davidson
Chairman, Working Group
December 1989

Contents

7

Tables

Figures

Introduction

1. At the meeting of the Scottish Health Service Planning Council on 16 June 1988, it was agreed that the Working Group on Prevention and Health Promotion be appointed, with the general terms of reference: 'To advise on health promotion and health education activities as requested by the Planning Council and the Scottish Home and Health Department'. The appointment of the Working Group endorsed the identification of prevention as a priority in both the SHAPE and SHARPEN reports[1,2].

2. The remit for the first of the series of tasks to be undertaken by the Working Group was: 'To review issues relating to the prevention of coronary heart disease, to examine activities undertaken by SHEG and health boards in this field, and to advise on a national approach to the prevention of coronary artery disease within which SHEG and health boards might operate'. A list of the members appointed to carry out this task is shown at Appendix 1.

3. In the course of its deliberations, the Group took evidence from a number of individuals and bodies whose details are given in Appendix 2. Visits were arranged to Good Hearted Glasgow, Be Better Hearted (Forth Valley), and Oxford Heart Attack and Stroke Prevention Project and Heartbeat Wales and a survey was conducted of relevant health promotion activities undertaken by health boards. Among material considered were the National Audit Office report, Coronary Heart Disease[3], the Consensus Statement of the King's Fund Forum on Blood Cholesterol Measurement in the Prevention of Coronary Heart Disease[4] and the Committee of Public Accounts report on Coronary Heart Disease[5], all of which were published in the course of the Group's life span. Members were also aware of the WHO Strategy Document, Health for All by the Year 2000, which set a minimum target of a 15% reduction in mortality from all diseases of the circulatory system[6].

4. Eight meetings were held, between October 1988 and November 1989. Two Sub-Groups were appointed in March 1989, to prepare recommendations on population and individual strategies.

5. The Working Group is grateful for the help and co-operation it received from persons giving evidence, arranging visits and participating in the survey.

Background

6. Scotland's unenviable record in heart disease mortality has been well documented[7,8]. Coronary heart disease (CHD) is the most common cause of death in Scotland, having accounted for 32% of all male deaths, and 26% of all female deaths, in 1988. (Figure 1 refers.) Its impact on middle aged men is particularly marked, around 40% of male mortality for 1988 in those aged 45–64 being attributed to this cause[9].

7. In addition to the social effects of premature deaths on surviving families, the costs to the NHS of treating CHD are considerable. In 1986, 400,000 hospital bed days in Scotland, at a cost of around £40,000,000, were occupied by patients with this condition[10,11].

8. The traditional view of the typical heart attack victim as an over-stressed senior executive no longer accurately reflects the social class distribution of coronary heart disease. As shown in Figure 2, the standard mortality ratio for this condition among men is now significantly higher for social class V than for the rest of the male population[12]. The figure also illustrates the increasing gradient, from 1970–72 to 1979–80/82–83, between men in social classes I, II and III non-manual and those in III manual, IV and V.

9. Comparisons with other countries, and an examination of trends over recent years, further underline the need for preventive action. The age-standardised mortality rates for thirty five countries, presented in an analysis of the latest available WHO data, published in 1988, show the Scottish female rate to be the highest recorded and the Scottish male rate to be exceeded only by Northern Ireland[13]. Although, as shown in Table 1, death rates for males in Scotland have fallen since the early 1970s, with the most marked decreases occurring in the youngest age groups, this downward trend has not matched the much more dramatic reductions which have been observed in some other countries[9,14]. (Figure 3 refers.)

10. It should be noted that although female rates of CHD are generally lower than those for males, a marked increase occurs in the former after the

menopause. As shown in Figure 4, the female rate for each 10 year age band over 45 is similar to, or above, the male rate for the preceding ten year band[10]. Moreover, deaths from CHD in women show even less of a downward trend than those in men. This is particularly evident in post-menopausal women in whom there has been little change in the past five years, Scottish women remaining at the top of the international league.

11. Although concerned primarily with the prevention of CHD, the Group was aware that, in addition to primary preventive measures, improvements in the diagnosis and treatment of angina pectoris, and myocardial infarction together with progress in cardio-pulmonary resuscitation (CPR), and secondary prevention would help reduce premature mortality from CHD[15]. Most deaths from heart attack occur outside hospital and the majority of these patients would respond to resuscitation. A growing public awareness of CPR may reduce the numbers of such deaths.

Coronary Heart Disease and Risk Factors

12. Coronary heart disease is caused by atherosclerosis of the coronary arteries in which deposition of lipid material stimulates the growth of smooth muscle, the production of fibrous tissue and the laying down of calcium in the wall of the artery. While this process may be diffuse throughout the arterial system, it is often accentuated in discrete areas known as plaques[16]. Typically, angina pectoris results from gradual narrowing due to plaque growth, while sudden death or myocardial infarction occurs when the plaque fissures, allowing blood to track behind it thereby further obstructing the vessel; the final event in total occlusion of the vessel is usually a blood clot (coronary thrombosis)[17].

13. The risk factor argument is based on the premise that a number of identifiable characteristics, some of which are reversible, are associated with an increased probability of CHD, and that the incidence of the disease can be reduced, or its onset delayed, by addressing these factors. This approach arises from extensive experimental epidemiological and clinical evidence[18, 19, 20]. The Group was aware of the professional debate about the use of the terms 'risk factor' and 'risk marker' in the context of a disease for which the cause or causes are incompletely understood, but agreed to use the first term since this is more widely accepted.

14. The relationship between CHD and the risk factors discussed below has been the subject of much debate in medicine. Within the Working Group a range of views existed on the extent to which specific risk factors had been shown conclusively to be related to the incidence and prevalence of CHD. It was nevertheless decided that the incidence of the disease could most effectively be addressed through this association.

(a) Non-reversible Risk Factors

15. The main non-reversible risk factors are age, male gender, a family history of premature CHD and diabetes. The presence of one or more

of these characteristics should not however be regarded as an inevitable harbinger of the development of CHD in an individual. Rather it should be taken as an indication of the need to employ preventive measures.

(b) Reversible Risk Factors

16. The major reversible risk factors are high blood cholesterol levels, smoking and high blood pressure, all of which interact synergistically to increase markedly the risk of CHD. This can be seen in Figure 5, taken from the MRFIT Study, in which the risk amplifying effect of cigarette smoking in subjects with and without high blood pressure and high cholesterol levels can be clearly seen[21]. Obesity and lack of physical exercise are also relevant risk factors.

(i) *High Blood Cholesterol*

17. High national rates of incidence of CHD occur in countries with high average levels of blood cholesterol, and rates are low where average cholesterol levels are low[22]. It has also been found that within populations, individuals who have high blood cholesterol levels are at greatest risk of developing CHD[23].

18. The process of atheroma formation, in which cholesterol plays a fundamental part, continues over many years prior to any clinical manifestations; the adverse effects of high blood cholesterol may therefore be regarded as a long term mechanism.

19. Individual levels of blood cholesterol can be influenced by the amount and ratio of polyunsaturated and saturated fats in the diet, and also to a lesser extent by smoking habits and the amount of physical exercise taken[24]. In addition, excessive blood cholesterol levels are found in a small proportion of people in whom it may be either familial or secondary to other diseases[25].

20. It is important to realise that cholesterol is an important component of all cells, and while high levels are associated with CHD, low levels have been found to be associated with cancer. This association is at least in part due to an effect of preclinical cancer on serum cholesterol levels[26].

21. The scope for tackling the incidence of CHD in Scotland through this risk factor is discussed later in the text. Some indication of this is given by a comparison of a generally acceptable adult level of 5.2 mmol/litre with the Scottish mean levels of 6.4 for males and 6.6 for females[27]. Studies have shown that a 1% fall in the cholesterol level of a population will result in a 2% fall in the incidence of CHD[28].

(ii) *HDL and LDL Cholesterol*

22. An individual's diet, smoking habits and exercise patterns affect the composition as well as the absolute level of his or her cholesterol, which is carried in the blood by lipoproteins with differing physical characteristics to which the terms high density (HDL), intermediate density (IDL) and low density (LDL) have been ascribed. The total level of cholesterol, as measured by conventional cholesterol testing, is the sum of these three fractions, with 60% to 70% being carried by the low density lipoproteins, and 20% to 30% by the high density lipoproteins.

23. The significance of the relative amounts of these lipoproteins lies in the perceived 'protective' property of HDL and the atherogenic potential of LDL. The amount of LDL in the circulating blood is affected by the activity of LDL 'receptors' in the liver whose function is to remove LDL from the blood. While the number and activity of these receptors is largely under genetic control, the blood levels of both LDL and HDL cholesterol can be influenced by behavioural factors. HDL cholesterol levels are increased by physical exercise and moderate alcohol intake, and decreased by smoking. LDL levels are increased by smoking and decreased by a reduction in the intake of saturated fat.

(iii) *Smoking*

24. Cigarette smoking is probably the most preventable of all the risk factors for CHD, and it has been estimated that 25% of all deaths from heart disease below the age of 65, and 50% of these in middle aged women are accounted for by smoking[28]. The spectrum of vascular disease associated with smoking includes not only CHD but also peripheral vascular disease and stroke; in addition smoking is the main cause of lung cancer, and contributes to the incidence of other conditions such as chronic respiratory disease. There is strong and unequivocal evidence that the incidence of and mortality from myocardial infarction increases progressively with the number of cigarettes smoked; a reversal of this trend accompanies cessation of smoking[22, 29].

25. The mechanisms underlying the association between smoking and CHD include damage to the endothelium (lining) of the blood vessel, a greater tendency for the blood to clot as a result of higher levels of fibrinogen (the precursor of fibrin, the main component of the clot itself), and increased stickiness of the blood platelets which initiate the formation of the clot[30].

26. Smoking levels in Scotland are among the highest in the UK, and are particularly high among women[9]. A disturbing proportion of school children, including those still attending primary school, also smoke. Smoking patterns

are affected both by educational awareness and by other, more complex factors. Messages about the adverse effects of smoking on health have been most readily received by Social Classes I and II, and it is likely that this has contributed to the differences in SMR between Social Classes referred to in paragraph 8. The majority of smokers have expressed the desire to stop[31].

(iv) *High Blood Pressure*

27. The link between high blood pressure and CHD is well established[32]; as with smoking, high blood pressure more than doubles the risk of CHD in those with high cholesterol levels. Abundant evidence also exists of other favourable results from lowering the blood pressure, including a reduction in the incidence of stroke, heart failure and renal failure[28].

28. The mechanism of the association between high blood pressure and CHD is unknown, and reducing the blood pressure with drugs may not decrease that risk[28]. High blood pressure is often associated with excessive energy intake resulting in obesity, and weight loss, which is now generally accepted as first line treatment for overweight patients, has a significant effect in lowering the blood pressure[33].

(v) *Physical Exercise*

29. The beneficial results of physical exercise, both physiological and psychological, are well documented. There are many reports claiming that it increases longevity and reduces coronary heart disease, but as yet, the evidence is such that these claims cannot be accepted unequivocally[34]. From a health promotion standpoint the most beneficial form of exercise involves large muscle groups in sustained rhythmical dynamic activity such as occurs during walking, running, dancing, swimming, cycling and other types of motion. Such activity is known as 'aerobic' because it requires a continuous supply of oxygen to and uptake by the exercising muscles. Other forms of exercise are predominantly anaerobic (without oxygen) and are characterised by short high intensity effort. Examples of this kind of activity are sprinting and weight lifting.

30. Aerobic physical training results in an increased uptake of oxygen during maximal exercise and therefore an enhanced physical work capacity. In practical terms the attainment of this 'cardiovascular fitness effect' means that for any given physical activity involving less than maximum effort, heart rate and blood pressure are lower than in untrained subjects. The circulation is therefore more efficient[35].

31. In addition to inducing improved mood and an enhanced feeling of well being, aerobic exercise contributes to the prevention of CHD through a decrease in resting blood pressure in both normal and hypertensive patients, an increase in HDL cholesterol and a reduction in body fat. It may also facilitate reduction in or cessation of cigarette smoking. Other beneficial effects include the prevention of osteoporosis in post-menopausal women and improved physical fitness in terms of suppleness, stamina and strength, depending on the type of activity undertaken[36].

32. In general terms, a significant training effect can be obtained by exercise which raises the resting heart rate to a level of resting heart rate plus 60% of the heart rate range* for 20 minutes at least three times a week[37]. It is recommended that this level of exercise participation be adopted as a target for all. Many types of physical activity, including numerous sports and games and even brisk walking, are suitable for the acquisition and maintenance of a cardiovascular training effect and its attendant benefits[38]. Advice on the activities most suited to or likely to be enjoyed by the individual should be more generally available, preferably by trained personnel in sports centres.

33. Results from the Scottish Heart Health Study, as shown in Table 2, indicate that a relatively small proportion of the Scottish population undertake regular exercise at the recommended level, and there is clearly a need to promote regular vigorous recreational activity as a lifetime commitment among young adults, with exercise programmes being tailored to suit the capabilities of participants. In subjects who have had heart attacks or bypass surgery, exercise is an important component of rehabilitation.

(vi) *Obesity*

34. The upper fifth of the distribution of obesity is associated with premature mortality, mainly due to coronary heart disease, but the risk of milder degrees of overweight is more controversial. Obesity may be an independent risk factor, or may exert its effect through hypertension, raised cholesterol levels or glucose intolerance[39].

(vii) *Stress*

35. Although stress is popularly believed to be related to coronary heart disease, the absence of an adequate definition frustrates its objective assessment. A study in this country showed an association between CHD (but not subsequent events) and Type A behaviour, which is characterised by, for instance, sustained aggression, ambition, competitiveness and a chronic

---

* The heart rate range is defined as 220 less age in years, less resting heart range.

sense of urgency[40, 41]. The WHO Expert Committee[42] noted that public and professional misconceptions about stress, whereby it is assigned a primary role in the genesis of coronary heart disease, may divert attention from demonstrated needs in prevention.

(viii) *Alcohol*

36. A link between heavy drinking and CHD has been described, although the often associated heavy cigarette smoking has made it difficult to confirm alcohol as an independent risk factor. Alcohol raises one fraction of the blood lipids, the triglycerides. Conversely, mild or moderate drinking has been claimed to be protective, by raising the levels of HDL cholesterol.

(c) **Prevalence of Risk Factors**

37. The Scottish Heart Health Study found that over two-thirds of respondents had at least one risk factor, and one fifth of both males and females had two risk factors. The prevalence of the major risk factors, ie blood cholesterol, smoking and high blood pressure, in the Scottish population, and the scope for its reduction, is shown in Table 3.

(d) **Action on Risk Factors**

38. Available evidence indicates that there is already a high level of public awareness of risk factors, of the prevalence of CHD as a major killer in Scotland, and of the behavioural modifications required to reduce the risk[43]. Although this knowledge has been translated into action by some individuals, notably members of Social Classes I and II, this has not been the case generally, and it is clear that the provision of information and advice alone is an inadequate educational tool with which to motivate all members of the public. The mechanisms by which this may be achieved are still the subject of research, but it is clear that strategies appropriate to the needs of Social Classes III, IV and V have yet to be developed.

39. The strength of the association between CHD and the major risk factors, cholesterol, cigarette smoking and high blood pressure, have led to a number of trials in which the effect of risk factor modification on subsequent CHD events was investigated. Exemplar trials in which one or more risk factors have been addressed are reviewed below.

(a) Single Risk Factor Intervention Studies

Cholesterol—Nutritional Change

40. It is difficult to change the diet of a given population in a precise way for long enough to produce meaningful results. Of particular interest, therefore, are studies in which institutionalised populations have undergone controlled nutritional change by catering interventions. The two studies most frequently quoted by prevention protagonists are the Los Angeles Veterans Study and The Finnish Mental Hospitals Study[44, 45]. In the Los Angeles trial, deaths due to CHD were not significantly reduced although deaths due to all 'atherosclerotic events' fell significantly by 31.3%; in the Finnish Study, CHD deaths were 53% lower in the diet as compared to the control groups. These results were associated with a significant reduction in serum cholesterol.

41. Both trials are flawed and at best it can only be considered that a favourable trend towards a fall in CHD mortality occurred. Benefit in total mortality cannot be claimed and in the Los Angeles Study (but not in the Finnish Study) there appeared to be an increase in non cardiac causes of death, especially cancer.

Cholesterol—Drug Treatment

42. Several trials have been reported, the two most recent and largest of which are the Lipid Research Clinics Trial which employed cholesturamine and the Helsinki Heart Study which used gemfibrozil[46, 47, 48]. Both these randomised controlled studies showed a significant reduction in coronary

events, although total mortality was unaffected due to an increase in deaths from other causes such as suicide and accidents. These results may be spurious but they recall the earlier Clofibrate Study which showed reduction in coronary events but an increased mortality in the intervention group due to an increase in deaths from cancer. Gallstones occurred more frequently in these drug trials.

Smoking

43. In the Whitehall Trial of British Civil Servants subjects were randomly assigned to a smoking cessation or a control group. At the end of 10 years there remained a 30% difference in smoking habit in the two groups and the CHD death rate was lower in the smoking cessation group[49]. Deaths from lung cancer fell, but to balance this there was an increase in non cardiac death especially non lung cancers. It is of interest that no further controlled trials of stopping smoking have been or are likely to be carried out in view of the obvious ethical issues raised by the widespread acceptance of the overall benefits of stopping smoking.

High Blood Pressure

44. This subject has been extensively reviewed recently[28]. Trials are consistent in finding a reduced incidence of stroke and heart failure. The Australian Trial and the Hypertension Detection and Follow Up Trial both found a reduction in deaths from CHD while in the latter Study, mortality from all causes was reduced by 17%. Although the more recent trials have been inconclusive in terms of CHD they have confirmed the marked decrease in stroke and heart failure seen in previous trials.

(b) **Multi-factorial Intervention Studies**

45. In the Oslo Primary Prevention Trial hypercholesterolaemic men (7–9.5 mmol/1), most of whom (70%) were smokers, were randomly allocated to an intervention group or to non intervention. Intervention consisted of advice on diet and stopping smoking. After five years there was a statistically significant reduction of 71% in sudden cardiac death and of 45% in CHD. Mortality from all causes was reduced by 31% which was not statistically significant[50].

46. The Multiple Risk Factor Intervention Trial (MRFIT) has been extensively discussed. Its results were disappointing because in the complete cohorts of subjects randomly allocated to special care (active intervention), and to usual care there was no significant difference in the primary end points. Risk

factors were reduced by both the special care group and the usual care subjects, and the net difference in risk factors between the two was smaller than expected[51].

47. Analyses of sub-groups must, necessarily, be treated with caution. However, those who were not hypertensive, and who were therefore very similar in their characteristics to those in the Oslo Trial, showed an equally striking reduction (49%) in CHD death rate[52]. Moreover, in subjects who had a positive exercise test for myocardial ischaemia (ie those with evidence of pre-existing CHD), CHD deaths were reduced by 63%[53].

48. In the WHO Collaborative Trial the results were not uniform in all participating countries. Deaths from CHD fell in Belgium, Italy and Poland and rose slightly in the UK[54]. In general, the reduction in risk from CHD was related to the extent of risk factor modification. For example, in the UK, which had the worst record for lowering risk factors, no significant change in CHD occurred. In Italy, where risk factor modification was greatest, a 28% reduction in CHD mortality took place, although this did not reach statistical significance.

49. In the Goteborg Trial, as in the MRFIT Study, both the intervention group and the control group reduced their risk factors significantly, and no difference in CHD or mortality was found between the two groups. It was concluded that a decrease in all three risk factors had taken place in the general population in Goteborg possibly as a direct consequence of the study[55].

50. The North Karelia Study compared two populations in Eastern Finland in one of which, North Karelia, active community intervention to reduce smoking, improve the diet and detect and treat hypertension was instituted[56]. After 10 years CHD mortality had declined by 24%. This reduction was significant when compared with the rest of Finland, but was not significantly greater than the slightly smaller decline in the reference area Kuopio. In women the more considerable decline in CHD mortality of 51% in North Karelia was significantly greater than in Kuopio. As in MRFIT and in Goteborg the population in the control group also significantly reduced their risk factors. The North Karelia Study highlights the difficulty of any form of controlled study in a population aware of the high risk of CHD and of the measures that might be taken to reduce that risk. In a subsequent communication one of the authors discussed these difficulties and pointed out that the fall in CHD in North Karelia may or may not have been the result of the prevention programme[57].

51. In some of these studies, the magnitude of the reduction in CHD was less than hoped for, suggesting that the educational aspects of risk factor change require further investigation. In addition each of the trials can be criticised on some aspects of design. But perhaps the most difficult issue in the context of advice to large populations is the indictment that none of them resulted in any decrease in total mortality. Perhaps the trials were neither large nor long enough, or the fall in risk factors great enough for this effect to be seen but most authorities accept that their effects on one or more of the common clinical manifestations of coronary heart disease were consistently favourable. The results of the trials are however consistent with the extensive clinical, pathological and epidemiological database concerning the major risk factors, indicating that their modification should form an important part of a community health strategy aimed at reducing premature death or disability from CHD.

Current Health Board Activities

52. Questionnaires were completed on behalf of each of the 15 Scottish health boards, giving information about boards' activities in the field of CHD prevention and also in other areas of health promotion such as nutrition and smoking, in September 1989.

53. At that time, four boards, Ayrshire and Arran, Dumfries and Galloway, Forth Valley and Greater Glasgow, reported CHD programmes in progress, two of which had been implemented in full and two in part. Of the remainder, one had a programme planned, but not yet implemented, five reported plans in preparation and five had no current plans for the introduction of a CHD programme.

54. Nutrition and smoking programmes had been introduced, in full or in part, in eight and 12 boards respectively, and were planned in all other boards with one exception. A relatively higher proportion of boards which did not intend introducing CHD programmes had implemented nutrition and/or smoking programmes. (Table 4 refers.)

55. Other non-disease specific programmes mentioned in responses included alcohol abuse (five boards), Look After Yourself (four boards) and other holistic initiatives (three boards).

56. Boards were invited to specify the goals of their CHD programmes, and six did so. Of these, three stated objectives relating to a reduction in morbidity and mortality, one was concerned with a reduction in risk factor related behaviour and two referred to both.

57. Two boards with CHD programmes reported problems in implementation, one citing opposition from advocates of a holistic approach, and the other reporting lower than expected levels of uptake and GP support. One board, with plans for a CHD programme in preparation, anticipated problems in obtaining finance and appropriate staff.

58. Although information was requested about annual budgets, actual or estimated, for health promotion programmes, this was not generally available, most boards stating that such initiatives were not separately costed. The four health boards with CHD programmes in progress were able to provide figures, but of the eight boards with nutrition programmes and the 12 with smoking programmes, only one of each gave an annual figure.

Health Promotion and Strategies for Prevention

(a) Health and Health Promotion

59. It is now generally accepted that improvements in health in most developed countries, including the UK, will be attained by the creation of environments which are conducive to good health and which encourage health-enhancing behaviour in individuals and communities. It is thus widely accepted that health promotion will be the principal method for achieving the World Health Organisation European Region's targets for health for all by the year 2000[58, 59].

60. The process of health promotion should be seen as attempting to maintain and improve health by encouraging individuals to adopt healthy lifestyles and also to create a healthy environment. The Working Group understood the concept of health promotion to include all measures which enhance well-being, prevent disease or disease progression, or enable patients to understand, come to terms with or manage their residual disability. Such measures include health education, national and local policies formulated to protect and improve health, and programmes designed to prevent ill health[60].

61. Since health is 'a state of complete physical, mental and social well-being and not merely the absence of disease or infirmity'[61], health promotion is concerned not only with altering individual lifestyles but also with encouraging changes to the social and physical environment. Because health and ill health are the products of a wide range of influences throughout society, health promotion and disease prevention can be satisfactorily achieved only with effective intersectoral collaboration. They are not the sole prerogative of designated health services.

62. The importance of involving the public in the achievement of public health has been widely acknowledged. Not only must the public become more involved in those activities which influence health, but the health services must become more responsive to the needs of the community they

are there to satisfy. A major role for health promotion activity is thus the raising of expectations, and the increased involvement of the public in health matters and health-related services[62].

63. Thus health promotion is concerned with:
a. Promoting a healthy environment;
b. Reducing preventable conditions;
c. Making healthy lifestyle choices available to individuals through education and the provision of services in the community;
d. Educating individuals towards better use of available services;
e. Ensuring that patients and their relatives are knowledgeable either about what is required for a restoration to former health, or how to make the most of their remaining potential for healthy living and how to avoid unnecessary hardships, restrictions and complications.

64. In general, health promotion operates at different levels, aiming to influence society and the environment, and assisting individuals to make informed choices about their health.

65. A recently developed model of health promotion which has been used widely was considered by the Group and was found to provide a useful framework for the task in hand[63]. This model identifies three components of health promotion: health education, defined as communication and activity aimed at enhancing well-being and preventing or diminishing ill health in individuals and groups; prevention, which is the reduction of risk of occurrence of a disease process, illness or some other unwanted event or state; and health protection, defined as legal or fiscal codes, other regulations or policies, or voluntary codes of practice aimed at the prevention of ill-health or the positive enhancement of well-being.

(b) **Strategies for Prevention**

66. Scotland has no national policy aimed specifically at the prevention of heart disease. Instead, a general, or holistic, approach has been adopted, promoting the concept of a healthy lifestyle. In preventive terms the reason for this is that the lifestyle practices associated with the incidence of CHD are also related to several other common preventable conditions such as stroke, lung cancer and chronic respiratory disease.

67. In terms of public education the national approach taken by the Scottish Health Education Group has been to inter-relate the individual issues of smoking, nutrition, exercise, alcohol abuse and others with campaigns

designed to promote general good health. For a number of years the integrating vehicle was a programme entitled 'Fit for Life' jointly mounted with the Scottish Sports Council. Since 1984 the vehicle has been 'Be All You Can Be'[64]. This approach was designed to help people accept that good health was enjoyable, that steps to achieve good health need not involve major changes in behaviour, and that the actions required in order to improve health could be made by all.

68. The Working Group accepted that promotion of a lifestyle which is in itself enjoyable and creates feelings of well-being is not only psychologically more likely to be acceptable but is entirely consistent with a broad understanding of health being more than the absence of disease. Lifestyle change which focuses on immediate benefits is likely to provide greater motivation for individuals and is also likely to provide a greater protective effect. A holistic approach allows for a wider range of lifestyle aspects which are related to health or a range of health problems to be dealt with. This is important since many aspects of lifestyle are clustered in terms of day to day living eg. smoking patterns and drinking behaviour. Holistic, broadly-based strategies are advocated by the WHO[65,66]. Members also recognised the need to improve the health of the Scottish population in general terms.

69. The respective merits of the holistic and disease specific approaches were considered at some length by the Working Group, and the latter was not recommended as a basis for public education, mainly on account of the overlap between the putative risk factors for CHD and other conditions. It was considered that the pursuit of a number of disease specific programmes would lead to duplication of effort and could result in confusing messages.

70. It was therefore recommended that a holistic strategy be adopted, incorporating a more robust and wider application of the principles contained in the Be All You Can Be programme[64]. They would consist of the provision of information and advice to members of the public on lifestyle patterns conducive to good health, and would be accompanied by action, involving the producers and suppliers of relevant goods and services, to facilitate the implementation of the advice provided. As far as possible, messages to the public would be framed in a positive manner, emphasising what should, rather than what should not, be done, in order to ensure optimum levels of acceptability. The proposed holistic strategy would result in the creation of an environment conducive to changes in lifestyle.

71. The Working Group however also agreed that in Scotland the prevention of CHD should be treated as a matter of priority. It was accepted that some

individuals were more susceptible to the condition because of identifiable factors such as high blood cholesterol, smoking, high blood pressure and a strong family history of CHD. While some of these factors would be susceptible to lifestyle change others would require general or specialist medical care. It was accordingly recommended that an assessment of CHD risk factors be undertaken to identify these individuals for whom more specific interventions or management strategies would be appropriate, in addition to general lifestyle advice consistent with the population approach. The approaches are thus complementary, the population strategy providing a backdrop against which it would become easier for individuals to respond to the advice they receive.

Recommended Action

72. This chapter describes the two strategies, population and individual, which the Working Group recommends should be implemented. Although these are treated separately, it will be seen that some degree of overlap, in both content and operation, is anticipated. The Group's recommendations on the evaluation of the combined programme is given in paragraphs 143 to 147.

73. Although it is expected that substantial savings in the cost of treating CHD and other conditions with the same risk factors would be achieved in the long term by the implementation of the Working Group's recommendations, some additional finance will be required for the programme. The Group was disturbed to learn of the relatively low priority currently accorded prevention and health promotion in Scotland. This is illustrated by a comparison of the amount spent on the 'Be All You Can Be' programme in 1987–88, which was identified by the Committee of Public Accounts as 14 pence per head of population, with the total cost of the NHS in Scotland for that year, around £550 per head[5]. Estimated costs and benefits are given in paragraphs 148 to 165.

74. The Group considered that the implementation and evaluation of a national health promotion policy would be effectively achieved only by a body of appropriate status and authority. It is therefore recommended that such a body, with responsibilities similar to that of the Health Education Authority in England, the Health Promotion Authority in Wales, and the Health Promotion Unit in Northern Ireland, be appointed, to operate in consultation with the Scottish Home and Health Departments and with a remit including relevant activities already undertaken by the Scottish Health Education Group, covering all health promotion topics. Such an organisation should participate in policy making and should have links with other appropriate Government Departments and agencies at national level. These links would facilitate the co-ordination necessary for the successful implementation of prevention programmes.

75. There is a need for central policy, along with guidance on implementation and evaluation, to be communicated to health boards: at the same time boards must be free to modify programmes and to set targets in the light of local circumstances. The CAMO of each board should be responsible for the preparation and implementation of local strategies and for inter-sector collaboration at local level with, for instance local authorities, whose co-operation is essential.

(a) The Population Strategy

76. The population strategy recognises that to a considerable extent the individual has the potential to control his or her lifestyle and thereby to influence his or her state of health. By encouraging members of the public to make choices which will result in a generally healthier lifestyle, it is intended to reduce coronary heart disease, and at the same time a number of other conditions such as stroke, chronic respiratory disease and lung cancer. The strategy encompasses education, to enable the right choices to be made; support, provided by health and other professionals; and measures to ensure that healthy choices are available to all who wish them. A co-ordinated approach, involving the health service, relevant Government Departments and other agencies, will be required for the effective implementation of this strategy.

77. The population strategy is directed towards the population as a whole, but should operate in parallel with the complementary strategy designed to meet the needs of those individuals who can be identified as likely to require a more personal form of intervention, as discussed in paragraphs 101 to 142.

78. Since it has been demonstrated that positive messages are more readily received than negative ones[67], the programme should concentrate on what should be done to improve health rather than on what should not be done, although it may be necessary at times to present negative messages in order to raise awareness. Another important educational principle is that benefits which allow individuals to enjoy life now should be stressed in favour of promises of future diseases to be avoided. The concept is particularly relevant in the case of those people likely to be most resistant to conventional health education programmes.

Programme Content

79. The three key elements of the population strategy are nutrition, which relates to three of the risk factors—cholesterol, hypertension and obesity—exercise and smoking, and although these are presented separately here, in

practice they will be integrated. There is a need for a national focus of expertise for each of the key elements of the programme, and it is recommended that these be established by the health promotion body referred to in paragraph 74, possibly in collaboration with existing institutions.

(i) Nutrition

80. Nutrition policies have been developed by various scientific expert committees for the prevention of cardiovascular disease[68] and for the wider prevention of non-communicable diseases[69]. A recent review of such developments throughout European countries has shown a remarkable uniformity in the content of national food and nutrition policies[70].

81. There is currently a lack of comprehensive data on Scottish nutritional patterns, although some information is provided by the National Food Survey and a small number of occasional surveys[62,70,71,72]. Such evidence as is available indicates that dietary habits fall short of these generally recommended, particularly in respect of a low intake of fruit, vegetables and wholegrain cereals, and excess fat and salt intake. Because of the crucial role which nutrition plays in shaping the health of a population, and because of its impact not only on heart disease but on a wide variety of chronic diseases ranging from dental caries to bowel cancer, it is clear that some action is now called for, both at national and local levels.

82. A suggested framework for a nutrition policy, based on the recent major reports[68,69,70], along with data on present nutrition in Scotland, are shown in Appendix 3 and it is recommended that within this framework more detailed guidelines be prepared, both for Scotland as a whole and for each health board area, by the body described in paragraph 74 and by CAMOs. The policy, and targets, require to be translated from nutrients into foods. This will require considerable expertise and will be a major educational undertaking.

83. The implementation of a nutrition policy will require the dissemination of information and advice, collaboration between relevant bodies, and the exploiting of the exemplar role of appropriate organisations such as the health service. By these steps it is hoped that knowledge about good nutrition will be accompanied by action, in for instance school and workplace catering.

84. Although dietary advice and education should be made generally available, the consumers most likely to benefit from it are school children, young people, young mothers who are still establishing their dietary patterns, and

groups who are known to have patterns very different from those recommended. Much of this educational work will require to be carried out with and through other agencies by personnel such as teachers, social workers and health visitors, and other target groups for education in nutrition policy include the food industry and health service professionals. The principles of healthy eating should be included in undergraduate medical education and student nurse training, and in post-qualification courses for all relevant staff.

85. From the consumer's viewpoint, a knowledge of those foods which together comprise a healthy diet is only part of the solution. The recommended foodstuffs should be available and attractively priced, and a uniform system of labelling should be introduced, presenting nutritional information in an acceptable and informative manner. Experience of the Heartbeat Wales project has shown that food manufacturers, producers, promoters and retailers can collaborate effectively with health promotion agencies in responding to, and encouraging consumer demands for 'healthy' foods[73]. The possibilities for similar collaboration in Scotland, on a wider scale than at present, should be explored.

86. At local level, community dietitians have a key role in establishing and implementing nutrition policies. They work with other professionals including those in primary care, community health projects, health education, social services and education. It is recommended that health boards should review community dietetic establishments as part of their health promotion strategy.

87. The proposed focus of nutritional expertise (paragraph 79) should undertake tasks such as the translation of nutritional advice into foods, the provision of advice to relevant bodies and individuals, guiding and supporting the work of community dietitians, liaison with the food industry, and evaluation and monitoring.

(ii) *Smoking*

88. It is recommended that the main features of the smoking policy should be discouraging children from starting to smoke, protecting non-smokers from the effects of passive smoking, and encouraging smokers to stop by providing help and support for those who wish to do so.

89. Since discouraging children and young people from starting to smoke is likely to be easier and more cost-effective than trying to help adults to stop, the former should be a key target group for this component of the population strategy. Because of current trends in smoking among school children, long

term strategies are required, to include the primary school age group, especially girls[74]. Programmes such as Smoke Busters[75], currently underway in a number of health boards, are to be encouraged because of their positive approach to non-smoking, but such programmes must be supported by the exemplar role of adults who are in a position to influence children's behaviour—parents, teachers and health professionals. It is clear that special efforts will be required among those population groups where levels of smoking among adults are high if the habit and its consequences are not to be perpetuated through succeeding generations, leaving an ever-widening gap between social classes.

90. In addition, the effective implementation of this part of the programme requires that the law in regard to the sale of tobacco to those under age should be effectively upheld, and that adequate measures be taken to protect children from the effects of tobacco advertising.

91. Although the right of individuals to choose to smoke must be preserved, there is a need to protect non-smokers from the effects of passive smoking. Smoking policies should ensure that the needs of both groups are met, by the banning of smoking in public or shared work areas, and the provision of designated smoking areas. Such policies have already been successfully implemented in a variety of settings, and their further adoption, by institutions, employers and those responsible for public services should be encouraged.

92. Surveys have shown that the majority of smokers would like to stop smoking and that each year a large proportion of smokers attempt to do so[31]. Breaking the habit can be difficult and although the counselling at present provided by GPs is effective, further support is needed in many cases. Help should be provided, by way of individual counselling or group support, for those who wish to stop smoking. Smoking cessation rates after one year using a number of different approaches range from 20% to 40%[76]. Appropriate support facilities should be developed for use under both the population and the individual strategies. (Paragraph 120 refers.)

93. Because of the importance of smoking as a central factor in those diseases that account for the majority of premature deaths in Scotland, new impetus should be given to the promotion of anti-smoking and smoking cessation initiatives. The proposed focus of expertise, to be developed by the health promotion body (paragraph 74) should draw on the experience of and collaborate with SHEG initiatives such as Glasgow 2000.

94. The implementation of a smoking policy requires commitment and action at many levels through a number of agencies. A key document is the report, Health Education in the Prevention of Smoking Related Diseases, published in 1983 by the Scottish Health Education Co-ordinating Committee[77] and endorsed by the Minister for Health and Social Work at the Scottish Office. This report made a number of detailed proposals about the implementation of a smoking policy and contained recommendations for UK Government Departments, the Scottish Home and Health Department, the National Health Service, Education and Local Authorities, the Health and Safety Executive, Employers' Associations, Trades Unions and Voluntary Organisations. These recommendations are still valid and should be implemented. A system for monitoring the extent and effects of implementation should also be established by the body described in paragraph 74.

(iii) *Exercise*

95. Exercise, in addition to being enjoyable, is relevant to the control of all three major risk factors—cholesterol, smoking and high blood pressure. Its promotion should therefore be given equal prominence to improvements in nutrition and the control of smoking.

96. The exercise policy should be based on the target level of participation described in paragraph 32. The success of this policy will depend on both the extent to which members of the public can be persuaded of the beneficial effects of regular physical exercise, and at the same time the provision of suitable facilities to allow such activities to take place. Collaboration continues to be required between the health service, at national or local level, and other agencies such as schools, the Sports Council, industry and community education. Community based exercise programmes, similar to that now operating in some boards, are to be encouraged, as is the Look After Yourself (LAY) programme[78]. (See paragraphs 139 and 140.)

97. The promotion of regular physical exercise to consumers is most likely to meet with success if the immediate benefits, such as the feeling of well being, the reduction in tension and depression and the social benefits of interaction with others, are emphasised, with information about other beneficial effects, as described in paragraph 32, also being made available. Advice about the physical demands, and the short and long term effects of different types of activity should be widely available, so that individuals can choose a suitable form of exercise. They should be encouraged to increase their participation to three times per week and to maintain it at that level.

98. Although some forms of exercise, such as walking, can be carried out without special facilities, requirements for other activities vary. It is important that recreational facilities of an appropriate standard should be accessible and economically available to all. Suitable space and equipment already exists in many schools and local authority premises, and health board initiatives, such as the opening up of facilities such as physiotherapy gymnasia, should be encouraged.

(iv) *Other Components of the Population Strategy*

99. Although alcohol has not been identified as an important risk factor for CHD, it is clear that drinking behaviour is related to leisure activities, dietary patterns and smoking behaviour, and should be considered as part of a healthy lifestyle programme. The Working Group endorsed the Scottish Health Education Co-ordinating Committee report, 'Health Education and the Prevention of Alcohol Related Diseases'[79].

100. Although stress was not found to be a major risk factor for CHD, coping with stress-related issues is a very important aspect of a lifestyle approach to health. Feelings of self-esteem, confidence and control are prerequisites for making decisions about health: stress-related feelings may present barriers for people who wish to act on advice provided by health professionals. In addition, stress-related problems are the cause of a significant number of visits to GPs. It is clear that the achievement of a positive attitude towards health or well-being is a worthy goal in its own right in terms of a healthy lifestyle.

(b) **The Individual Strategy**

101. The individual (high risk) strategy is recommended by the Working Group for those at greatest risk of developing clinical manifestations of, or dying prematurely from CHD, and also for the disadvantaged, who are less likely than other groups to respond to health promotion messages. By focusing on high risk individuals the strategy attempts to promote lifestyle changes through the provision of advice on personal targets and their attainment.

102. There are two components to the strategy—the identification, by assessment or other means, of people at high risk, and the provision on an individual basis, of advice, treatment and follow-up as appropriate. Both are discussed below.

103. The overall responsibility for the implementation of the individual prevention strategy should rest with health boards, and the CAMO should

be responsible for the planning, promotion and co-ordination of assessment programmes in each board. Although, as noted below, much assessment and follow-up counselling can be carried out using existing resources, it will be necessary for some boards to demonstrate their commitment to the reduction of CHD, by the allocation of additional staffing resources, the amount of which will depend on the extent of current work and on the distribution of risk factors in each board's area.

104. Several mechanisms through which the strategy might be operated exist, or could be established. In view of the growing emphasis on health promotion in general practice, the support expressed for this in the White Paper, Working for Patients, and the Working Group's conviction that primary care provides the most effective channel for communications to patients, it is recommended that the strategy be based on the primary care system as is the case with other screening programmes, such as cervical cytology.

105. In making this recommendation, the Working Group recognises that commitment to the programme on the part of GPs will be crucial to its success, and recommends that every effort be made to enlist their support.

Target Population for Assessment

106. High risk individuals can be identified in two ways. Firstly, an examination of primary care practice records can identify those with a previous history of CHD, and those already known to have risk factors. Secondly, risk factors should be identified by an opportunistic assessment programme. The Working Group considered that those in the age group 35–60 would be most receptive to, and therefore most likely to benefit from this approach.

107. With at least one third of heart attacks occurring in patients already known to have CHD, a previous history of the disease is the strongest of all risk factors[80]. It is also known that such patients accept and adhere to lifestyle changes and that such action is effective in reducing recurrent CHD[32, 81]. The expense incurred by the NHS in the acute management of such patients is considerable, and in order to maximise the return on this investment, post-discharge support is essential. It is recommended that all patients with evidence of CHD such as angina, and those who have had myocardial infarctions, coronary bypass grafts or angioplasty be included among those to be assessed. Since responsibility for such patients is shared between primary care and hospital services, care must be taken to avoid duplication of effort between the two.

36

108. It is already considered good practice for patients' risk factors to be recorded by GPs along with other aspects of their medical history, and a considerable proportion of patients with risk factors can be readily identified. For some of these a full risk factor profile will already be available: others will require further assessment.

109. It is clear that CHD is more prevalent among those in social classes IV and V. (Paragraph 8 refers.) Detailed and accurate information on nutrition by social class is not available, but cigarette smoking and a lack of leisure time exercise are features of groups IV and V[82]. It must be acknowledged that the perception of need in such groups differs widely from that of those usually responsible for service planning. This is sometimes reflected in the under use of facilities which have been provided.

110. The target population for assessment among socially disadvantaged groups will require to be defined locally. Other groups who may need special consideration include ethnic communities such as Asians, among whom the incidence of CHD is high[83].

Programme Content–Assessment

111. It is recommended that the assessment programme should be based upon the three main risk factors—high blood cholesterol, smoking and high blood pressure—and also physical exercise and obesity. Criteria for intervention, by risk factor, are shown in Appendix 4. Assessment should be accompanied by the provision of lifestyle advice, which would reinforce the messages of the population strategy.

112. The desirability of the mass measurement of cholesterol levels, which is advocated in the United States and elsewhere, and which is currently the subject of wide debate in the UK, was considered by the Study Group. It was accepted that knowledge of their cholesterol levels might enhance the motivation of those individuals likely to benefit from dietary and other changes, although data on this effect are not yet available. On the other hand, awareness of levels might induce anxiety in some and complacency, both equally unwarranted, in others. Furthermore, the high average level of the Scottish population would result in a considerable number of individuals being found to have cholesterol levels which are unacceptably high, suggesting that dietary and other advice provided generally might be a more cost-effective way of addressing the probelm.

113. Some concern has been expressed over recent developments in the provision of cholesterol measurement. Until now, this has been carried out,

in the majority of cases, in laboratories, and the results have not been available to patients at the initial consultation. Desk top devices are now being used to a growing extent but it has been found that they are prone to operator faults[84, 85].

114. Following its deliberations on the arguments for and against measuring cholesterol levels in the population, the Working Group concluded that cholesterol screening should be restricted to those most likely to benefit from it. It is therefore recommended that cholesterol measurement should be carried out in respect of those among the assessment population who have recognised vascular disease, or a history of premature CHD (before the age of 50) or of hyperlipidaemia in a first degree relative. This recommendation broadly endorses the findings of the recent King's Fund Consensus Development Conference on Cholesterol Measurement[4].

115. Blood pressure should be measured in accordance with available guidelines[86], and patients with diastolic levels above 95 mm Hg should be identified as requiring advice or treatment. High blood pressure is likely to be accompanied by reversible factors such as obesity, excess alcohol consumption, poor physical fitness, excess salt intake, and possible environmental stress.

116. Advice and/or treatment as appropriate should be given to all those whose cholesterol is measured and is found to be over 5.2 mmol, smokers, those with diastolic blood pressures above 95 mm Hg, those who do not regularly reach exercise target levels (see paragraph 32) and persons who are obese, ie whose weight is at least 20% above the normal for their height and sex.

Advice and Treatment

117. The recommended intervention for patients identified through the assessment programme as being at risk is described below in general terms, and shown in greater detail in Appendix 4.

(i) *High Blood Cholesterol*

118. Nutritional counselling, on an individual basis, incorporating advice on weight loss and smoking where appropriate, should be provided initially, by staff involved in assessment, to those with high cholesterol levels, with the exception of persons with levels greater than 10 mmol, who should be referred to lipid clinics. Drug therapy may ultimately be considered appropriate for persons with persistently high cholesterol levels, but should be prescribed only following full investigation, taking into account all the relevant clinical

circumstances, and after nutritional and lifestyle advice has proved unsuccessful. Drugs should not normally be prescribed for people with levels below 10 mmol.

119. It should be noted that because of the significant increase in cholesterol levels in post-menopausal women, counselling is likely to be required in respect of a large number of such patients.

(ii) Smoking

120. As noted in paragraph 92 mechanisms to help smokers break the habit should be developed for use under both the population and the individual strategies. All smokers should be advised to stop, and those who wish to do so should be given individual counselling to be followed, if required, by participation in a stop smoking group. Alternative techniques such as the use of nicotine chewing gum, acupuncture and hypnotherapy have all been tried but efficacy has been poorly substantiated[76].

(iii) High Blood Pressure

121. Some patients will reduce their blood pressure to an acceptable level by following lifestyle advice. Others will require drug treatment, the guidelines and special facilities for this being already well established. Recommendations on intervention are given in Appendix 4.

122. In cases where excessive consumption of alcohol accompanies high blood pressure appropriate advice should be provided. GPs are well placed to detect and counsel heavy drinkers, and there is evidence that this can be effective[87].

(iv) Physical Exercise

123. Individuals whose level of physical activity is below the desired level should be advised of the benefits of fitness and encouraged to take up exercise. (See paragraph 32). The acceptability of such advice will to some extent be determined by the success of the population approach, which should promote the development of exercise facilities within the community.

(v) Obesity

124. Reduction of excess body weight lowers blood pressure and serum cholesterol, and reduces the every day work of the heart, in addition to improving the body image. Obese individuals should be advised on weight loss and encouraged to participate in local support groups where these exist; primary care teams in larger practices or health centres might consider

setting up such groups. In special circumstances, such as severe obesity and hypercholesterolaemia, direct counselling by dietitians will be necessary. Such staff should also be encouraged to contribute to the prevention of CHD by advising and training other health professionals in appropriate dietary strategies.

Follow-Up

125. The follow-up of patients with risk factors fulfils two functions—the monitoring of progress towards individual targets and the reinforcement of advice provided at initial assessment sessions. While it can be argued that patients who smoke, and those who are obese, should be able to monitor their own progress, some of these will need additional counselling, accompanied where available by practical assistance. Not all of those who require such help will seek it, and it is therefore recommended that an appropriate follow-up system be established in each practice.

126. In the case of patients with high blood pressure and/or high cholesterol levels, whether or not other risk factors are also present, feedback is essential in order to monitor progress. Those with excessively high levels of blood pressure or cholesterol are identified in Appendix 4 as requiring immediate treatment initially at least by the GP. Others, with moderately high levels, should be invited to attend a follow-up session as appropriate, in order to assess the effectiveness of the advice provided and the patient's compliance with it.

127. At the follow-up stage it will be possible to identify those patients whose conditions have improved and who will not require further advice, those who have failed to accept the advice provided and for whom further counselling is unlikely to be appropriate, and those who appear to have complied with the advice given them but who require further treatment. This last group should be referred as appropriate.

Implementation

(i) *The Primary Care Team*

128. Those already known to have risk factors (see para 106), persons with a history of CHD, and other relevant groups will be readily identifiable from practice records. In the case of the remainder of the 35–60 age group, risk factors may be detected opportunistically when the patient presents for any reason or through routine contact with the primary care team.

129. In many practices, patients' blood pressure is already measured, their smoking status established and the relevant details of family history recorded in the patient records, with the GP himself undertaking assessment and counselling as well as the provision of treatment: except in a few areas, no systematic follow up is carried out. In busier urban practices such health promotion activities are more difficult to carry out and, depending on the area, the population may not be receptive.

130. A systematic approach is clearly required, in order to ensure that all patients within the recommended target groups are given the opportunity of assessment, and, where appropriate, adequate follow-up is provided. The new GP contract encourages this development. It is known that some 90% of individuals attend their GPs on at least one occasion in every five years, and the offer of a health check can be made in the course of a routine appointment.

131. It is recommended that in each practice, a designated person, who will normally be a nurse, be responsible for ensuring that appropriate patients are identified and offered assessment, that an assessment system once set up, is satisfactorily operated, and that follow-up appointments are arranged and referrals made.

132. It has been estimated that the assessment of the target population, if spread over five years, would in the case of some practices amount to one session per week, and could be absorbed by existing nursing staff: in others, new appointments will be necessary. But before these are considered, an attempt must be made to ensure that existing nurse staffing resources are fully utilised. The health promotion role of the health visitor, whose potential contribution to this programme may be impeded by current organisational constraints, should not be overlooked. Health visitors, whose broad training is particularly relevant to this work, have been successfully employed in Good Hearted Glasgow, although for administrative and practical reasons some GPs prefer to utilise the services of a practice nurse, as in the Oxford project[88]. As a significant number of sessions will be required overall in Scotland the financial implications of the grading of this nurse could be sizeable.

133. Experience to date suggests that in some boards the development of assessment programmes would be assisted by the employment of a facilitator, who would promote the programme among primary care teams, train the nursing staff and monitor progress. Such posts, which are based on the Oxford model, are generally held by health visitors[88].

134. The introduction of the programme should be phased, focusing initially on those known to be at greatest risk. Following the systematic selection and assessment of patients known by the general practitioner to be at increased risk, either through health-related risk factors or social circumstances, opportunistic screening of the remainder of the practice should take place. By this time, the various group sessions for anti-smoking advice, weight control and exercise should be established.

135. Consideration should be given to the timing of assessment sessions and follow-up appointments, in order to maximise uptake.

136. The further use of the GPASS system will facilitate the identification of patients at risk, to be assessed or requiring follow-up. This system is likely to become available to all primary care teams by mid-1991, and as a result of current developments will become easier to use. It is recommended that existing software, as used in breast cancer screening, be modified by the addition of an assessment capability, enabling it to be used, along with existing hardware, in this programme.

(ii) *Alternative Assessment Mechanisms*

137. Some high risks people will remain undetected, either because they do not visit their GPs or because they fail to accept the offer of a health check. For such people, who are likely to include those from disadvantaged communities, the reasons for non-participation should be explored, and health boards should take the initiative and arrange other opportunities for assessment. In order to ensure that such mechanisms are effective, however, it is essential that details of test results be communicated to GPs.

138. Assessment could be offered, by arrangement with employers, in the workplace: drop in centres could be established in settings such as town halls, supermarkets and sports centres: and mobile teams, providing both assessment and follow-up counselling, could operate in areas where the caseload is high or where the local practice provision is sub-optimal because of lack of premises or commitment.

(iii) *Support Groups*

139. In addition to, or as an alternative to counselling groups set up to provide advice and support to patients on specific risk factors, the Look After Yourself! (LAY) project, which was developed as a preventive measure by the Health Education Authority, and which is now under review, offers a holistic programme to groups of patients[78]. The programme is run by qualified

trainers, and consists of ten sessions, covering exercise, relaxation and several other health related topics such as nutrition and stress.

140. A report by the University of Nottingham found the LAY scheme to be successful in promoting behaviour modifications in those who wished to make informed choices about all aspects of their lifestyles through self-awareness[89]. It has been adopted by several health boards in Scotland.

(iv) Workload Implications

141. It should be noted that the recommended assessment programme will lead to a considerable increase in the workload of GPs and also in referrals to specialist facilities. There will also be a demand for additional training among primary care and other staff, and for health promotion material.

142. In addition, a greater awareness of risk factors such as high blood cholesterol among members of the public, arising from the population strategy, will inevitably result in some additional workload for GPs and laboratory staff.

Evaluation

143. It is recommended that a formal evaluation system should be developed for the programme, in order to assess both the feasibility of its strategies and its performance against objectives, long and short term. Where boards have already set up CHD prevention programmes, these should be evaluated. Some have recently initiated their own evaluation arrangements: others should be encouraged to do so.

144. A specific objective of the programme is the reduction of both incidence of and premature mortality from CHD. These are long term goals, on which progress can be monitored through data available from the Registrar General, Scotland, and from agencies such as the MONICA project[78]. The monitoring of costs and outputs, which will be necessary in order to ensure the effective deployment of resources in the shorter term, may be achieved by the adoption of a number of surrogate measures, such as patterns in risk factor behaviour.

145. Appropriate objectives—biological, behavioural, attitudinal and pertaining to service provision—must be defined and targets set by the body referred to in paragraph 74, in collaboration with health boards where relevant. Much baseline information on these is already available from SHEG and other sources: standardised follow-up surveys will be necessary. There is for instance evidence that the components of a healthy lifestyle are generally well understood by members of the public.

146. In addition to evaluating overall progress for Scotland and for individual health board areas, the collection of information should help to ensure that health promotion resources are being optimally distributed, both geographically and also between the two components of the programme. The evaluation of the population strategy, for instance, requires not only that changes in behaviour and knowledge be measured, but also that the effectiveness of the strategy's messages be assessed. This can be achieved by the use of some

of the sophisticated market research techniques developed by the advertising industry.

147. The success of the programme will be affected to some extent by external factors, which are outwith its control. Ultimately a system of environmental monitoring should be developed, in order to assess the impact of these.

Financial Implications

148. For a variety of reasons it has not been possible to carry out a full cost-benefit assessment of the recommendations set out in this report. Much of the information required for such an appraisal is not available. An attempt has been made, however, to identify the nominal costs and to illustrate the potential economic benefits that could be associated with an effective health promotion and prevention strategy.

149. The figures shown below need to be interpreted with some care. In the case of costs, for instance, the Working Group was aware that some screening and follow-up is already taking place in Scotland. Since little information on the extent of this is available, it proved impossible to take account of it in the calculations, and as a result the costs shown represent the total expenditure which would be necessary if no such initiatives were already under way.

150. In addition, it should be noted that costs would be incurred in the short term, whereas it would take some time for the full economic benefits to be achieved. Because of uncertainty about the timescale of the latter, no attempt has been made to discount the benefits.

151. In the case of savings, it should be noted that the estimates do not imply that in the longer term it will be possible to reduce expenditure on the NHS. Resources currently used for the treatment of CHD and other diseases will—if the strategy is effective—be released and be available for use elsewhere within the NHS. In so far as people live longer as a result of a reduction in, say, CHD, they are likely to require treatment for other age-related conditions at a later stage in their life and thus will obviously require extra resources.

152. The Working Group recommends a programme based on both a population and an individual approach, and no attempt has been made to relate potential savings to particular approaches. Although it is not possible at this stage to assess the relative effectiveness of different aspects of the strategy, this is an issue which will require careful evaluation.

(a) Costs

153. The individual strategy involves an initial assessment of patients and a series of follow-up measures directed at high risk individuals. It is proposed that the initial assessment of patients would be carried out at GP surgeries by nursing staff and would take an estimated 20 minutes per patient. It is recommended that all members of the target population be offered assessment over a five year period and that uptake will be around 75%. The estimated total cost of this initial screening would be around £600,000 per annum but it should be noted that, in an average list size of 2,000 patients, two or three persons per week would require assessment, and this work would not, in many cases, incur additional expenditure. The annual cost would be reduced after five years since maintenance assessment only would be required thereafter. The costs of follow-up involve the further treatment of three risk factors: smoking, cholesterol and high blood pressure. The method used to assess cases is as follows:—

Smoking

Additional counselling of heavy smokers by nursing staff and GPs would cost around £500,000 per year.

High Blood Pressure

Patients identified as having high blood pressure will be given nutritional counselling. Some may require drugs, and the annual cost of these measures excluding the cost of drugs already prescribed, has been estimated at £400,000.

Cholesterol

Dietary advice will be appropriate for many patients with raised cholesterol levels. Drugs will be required for a small proportion. If the use of drugs is confined to patients with cholesterol levels over 10 mmol the cost will be £3 million pa. Costs will however escalate rapidly if drugs are more widely prescribed. For instance, the cost of treating all patients with cholesterol levels over 8 mmol with drugs would be £40 million pa.

154. The total cost of the individual strategy would be:—

Initial Screening	£600,000
Follow-up:	
Smoking	£500,000
High Blood Pressure	£400,000
High Blood Cholesterol	£3,000,000–£40,000,000
Total	£4,500,000–£41,500,000

155. Drug costs for cholesterol represent a major part of the overall costs and clearly this item could be very expensive. The Group emphasised that the most appropriate method of lowering cholesterol is by nutritional change and that drugs should not be seen in any way as a substitute. Quite clearly the best protection against inappropriate prescribing will be the availability at all levels of patient contact of suitable nutritional advice and counselling. In the absence of a system incorporating selective testing and nutritional counselling, costs could be difficult to control.

156. No attempt has been made to estimate the costs of the population strategy. Further work will require to be carried out on this once the details of its various components have been finalised. There might be some merit in examining the costs of bodies such as Heartbeat Wales.

(b) Benefits

157. An effective strategy for health promotion and prevention should give rise to a number of important economic benefits. First, it should lead to a saving in the costs to the health service of treating CHD and other diseases with similar risk factors (cancer of trachea, bronchus and lung, cerebrovascular disease, bronchitis and other diseases of the circulatory system). In 1986 patients with these diseases spent 2.1 million days in hospital. Just over 1 million of these in-patient days can probably be attributed to the specific risk factors of smoking, cholesterol and high blood pressure—this is equivalent to around 4,000 hospital beds.

158. The average cost of in-patient care in an acute hospital currently averages £100 per day. The total costs of in-patient care attributed to risk factors is about £100 million. Out-patient services probably add a further £20 million giving a total hospital cost of £120 million. New and improved procedures for the treatment of heart disease such as coronary artery bypass grafts and angioplasty are expensive, and the costs of treating patients suffering from CHD is likely to rise as these procedures become more widely used.

159. In addition, CHD and other diseases related to the same risk factors give rise to significant costs in the General Practitioner Services. In 1986, expenditure on drugs related to this group of diseases came to almost £51 million. Again about 50% of this, some £26 million, can probably be related to the specific risk factors of smoking, cholesterol and high blood pressure. The cost to primary care of consultations for the above conditions is unknown, but is likely to cost at least £5 million pa. If half of this sum is attributed to risk factors, this would imply a cost of £2.5 million.

160. The costs to the NHS of treating the diseases directly related to smoking, cholesterol and high blood pressure in 1988–89 are summarised below:

	£m
Hospital	120.0
Pharmaceutical	27.0
General Practice	2.5
Total	148.5

161. There are wider economic costs to consider. CHD and other diseases impose a cost through absenteeism from work. In addition premature deaths among people of working age involve a substantial loss of output. Again it is difficult to quantify and value these effects accurately, but the following estimate may give a useful indication of the substantial economic costs involved.

162. In 1988–89 there were 11.1 million days of certified incapacity among people suffering from CHD, cancer of trachea, bronchus and lung, cerebrovascular disease, bronchitis and other diseases of the circulatory system. The value of this lost output was £450 million. Again, about 50% of this can probably be attributed to the specific risk factors of smoking, cholesterol and high blood pressure.

163. At present, the extent to which the proposed health promotion and prevention strategy will lead to a reduction in the incidence of CHD and other diseases is very uncertain. The following table shows the resource savings that could be obtained under a range of different assumptions about the reduction in the incidence of diseases directly related to smoking, cholesterol and high blood pressure.

	Estimated costs	Potential savings in costs		
	£m	Reduction of 10% £m	Reduction of 25% £m	Reduction of 50% £m
NHS costs	150	15	38	75
Lost output through certified incapacity	450	45	112	225
Total	600	60	150	300

164. A reduction of 10% in the incidence of diseases related to the relevant

49

risk factors would produce an annual saving of £60 million. A 50% reduction would produce an annual saving of £300 million. (These figures do not include any economic savings through a reduction in premature deaths among people of working age).

165. The purpose of this section of the report is to identify the economic costs and benefits of a programme of health promotion and prevention. This analysis is not intended to imply that the case for adopting such a programme should rest largely on narrow economic arguments. While it is important that we should be aware of the economic implications, the case for adopting the recommendations should be seen largely in terms of the contribution they can make to extending people's lives and improving the quality of their lives.

(c) *Alternative Sources of Funding and Commercial Activities*

166. Although additional funding will be required to set up the proposed CHD prevention programme, there appears to be a number of opportunities for commercial activities or alternative funding of specific initiatives once the programme has been established.

167. It is recognised that practical problems relating to this area, and the risk of compromise to the programme's messages, must be overcome before this can be a feasible option. Nevertheless, given the general level of interest in health which exists in Scotland, it is likely that a considerable contribution towards the programme's running costs might be met from, for instance, commercial sponsorship of special events, fund raising by voluntary bodies, and sales of attractively designed promotional material, including videos produced in collaboration with television companies.

168. An individual CHD screening package could be developed for industry, with the secondary aim of helping employers reduce levels of sick absences relating to CHD risk factors. A fee would be payable for each employee screened. The package would require to make provision for follow-up as necessary, through repeat visits of screening staff, the company doctor or occupational health nurse, or the patient's own GP.

169. On a local basis, initiatives such as the opening of appropriate health board premises to the general public, and the provision of Look After Yourself courses as part of general adult education programmes, might also be operated on a commercial basis.

170. Other possibilities include the commercial development of packages in fitness testing/exercise programmes, cardio-pulmonary resuscitation and

exercise in the workplace, the secondment of staff from commerce, and the achieving of Charitable Trust status, with resulting benefits in investment income and spending power. Additional funding may also be available from EEC sources, and through research grants.

Recommendations

1. A holistic population approach should be adopted. This should be complemented by an assessment programme which would identify high risk individuals and at the same time provide general advice and counselling. (Paragraphs 70, 71)

2. A national health promotion body, with responsibilities similar to those of the corresponding bodies in England, Northern Ireland and Wales, should be appointed for Scotland. (Paragraph 74)

3. The CAMO of each health board should be responsible for the preparation and implementation of local strategies and for inter-sector collaboration at local level. (Paragraph 75)

The Population Strategy

4. A co-ordinated approach, involving the health service, relevant Government Departments and other agencies is required for the effective implementation of the population strategy. (Paragraph 76)

5. The population strategy, covering nutrition, smoking and exercise, should be communicated by means of positive messages, and should concentrate on immediate benefits. (Paragraphs 78, 79)

6. The proposed Scottish health promotion body should establish foci of expertise in respect of the three key elements of the population programme. (Paragraph 79)

7. Detailed guidelines on nutrition, based on recent reports, should be prepared nationally for Scotland and locally for each health board area. (Paragraph 82)

8. The nutrition policy should be implemented by means of the dissemination of information and advice to consumers, collaboration between the relevant bodies, and the exploiting of the exemplar role of appropriate organisations. (Paragraph 83)

9. The dissemination of nutritional advice should be carried out by appropriate staff in a number of different agencies: it should be directed towards consumers, the food industry and health service professionals. (Paragraph 84)

10. The principles of healthy eating should be included in undergraduate medical education and student nurse training, and in post-qualification courses for all relevant health service staff. (Paragraph 84)

11. Recommended foodstuffs should be available, attractively priced and properly labelled. (Paragraph 85)

12. The possibilities of increased collaboration between health promotion agencies, at national and local levels, and the food industry should be explored. (Paragraph 85)

13. Health boards should review the establishment of community dietitians. (Paragraph 86)

14. The smoking policy should discourage children from starting to smoke, protect non-smokers from the effects of passive smoking, and encourage and help smokers to stop. (Paragraph 88)

15. Education on smoking should start in primary schools. Special efforts will also be required among population groups with high levels of smoking among adults. (Paragraphs 89)

16. The law in respect of the sale of tobacco to those under age should be effectively upheld. (Paragraph 90)

17. Adequate measures should be taken to protect children from the effects of tobacco advertising. (Paragraph 90)

18. Smoking policies should ensure that the needs of both smokers and non-smokers are met. (Paragraph 91)

19. Smokers who wish to stop should be given help, through individual counselling or group support. (Paragraph 92)

20. Support facilities for those who wish to give up smoking should be developed for use under both the population and the individual strategies. (Paragraphs 92, 120)

21. The recommendations made in the report, Health Education in the Prevention of Smoking Related Diseases, should be implemented. (Paragraph 94)

22. The exercise policy should be based on the recommended level of physical exercise. (Paragraphs 32, 96)

23. Collaboration in respect of the implementation of the exercise policy will be required between the health service, local authorities and other appropriate agencies. (Paragraph 96)

24. Advice about the demands and effects of different types of activity should be widely available. (Paragraph 97)

25. Recreational facilities of an appropriate standard should be accessible and economically available to all. (Paragraph 98)

26. Alcohol and stress should be included in the population strategy, as part of a healthy lifestyle programme. (Paragraph 99)

The Individual Strategy

27. The overall responsibility for the implementation of the individual strategy should rest with health boards. (Paragraph 103)

28. The CAMO in each board should be responsible for the planning, promotion and co-ordination of assessment programmes. (Paragraph 103)

29. The individual strategy should be based on the primary care system, and every effort should be made to enlist the support of GPs. (Paragraphs 104, 105)

30. The strategy should focus, for assessment purposes, initially on persons who have a previous history of heart disease, and those who are known to have risk factors. In addition, other high risk individuals should be identified by means of an opportunistic assessment programme directed towards the 35 to 60 age group. (Paragraph 106)

31. Assessment should be based on risk factors, and should be accompanied by lifestyle advice. (Paragraph 111)

32. Cholesterol measurement should be restricted to those with recognised vascular disease, and those with a family history of premature CHD or of hyperlipidaemia. (Paragraph 114)

33. Blood pressure should be measured in accordance with available guidelines. (Paragraph 115)

34. All persons found to have blood cholesterol levels above 5.2 mmol, smokers, those with diastolic blood pressures above 95mmHg, persons not regularly attaining the target for physical exercise and those who are obese should be given appropriate advice and/or treatment. (Paragraph 116, Appendix 4)

35. Persons with blood cholesterol levels between 5.2 and 10.0 mmol should initially receive nutritional and lifestyle counselling: those with levels over 10.0 should be referred to lipid clinics. (Paragraph 118, Appendix 4)

36. Lipid lowering drugs, which may be considered appropriate for persons with persistently high blood cholesterol levels, should be prescribed only after a full investigation, and after nutritional and other lifestyle advice has proved unsuccessful. Drugs should not normally be prescribed for persons with levels below 10 mmol. (Paragraph 118)

37. All smokers should be advised to stop. Those who require additional help, should be given individual counselling, followed, if required, by participation in a stop smoking group. (Paragraph 120)

38. Where lifestyle advice fails to achieve acceptable levels of blood pressure, drug treatment should be provided. (Paragraph 121, Appendix 4)

39. In cases of excessive consumption of alcohol, especially where this is accompanied by high blood pressure, appropriate advice should be given. (Paragraph 122)

40. Individuals whose level of physical activity is below the recommended level should be advised of the benefits of fitness and encouraged to take up exercise. (Paragraph 123)

41. Obese individuals should be advised on weight loss and encouraged to participate in support groups. (Paragraph 124)

42. Dietitians should be encouraged to advise and train other health professionals in appropriate dietary strategies. (Paragraph 124)

43. Appropriate follow-up systems should be established in each GP practice (Paragraph 125)

44. A designated person in each practice, normally a nurse, should be responsible for the operation of the assessment programme. (Paragraph 131)

45. Before new appointments are made, an attempt must be made to ensure that existing nurse staffing resources are fully utilised. (Paragraph 132)

46. The introduction of the assessment programme should be phased, concentrating initially on those who are known to be at greatest risk. (Paragraph 134)

47. Following the completion of current developments of the GPASS system, existing software should be modified by the addition of an assessment capability, enabling it to be used along with existing hardware, in the assessment programme. (Paragraph 136)

48. Alternative assessment mechanisms should be introduced where appropriate. The results of individuals' tests should be communicated to their GPs. (Paragraph 137)

Evaluation

49. A formal system of evaluation should be established for all aspects of the programme, in order to assess the feasibility of its strategies and its performance against objectives. (Paragraphs 143 to 147)

50. Boards with CHD prevention programmes already in operation should be encouraged to evaluate them. (Paragraph 143)

References

1. Scottish Home and Health Department. Scottish Health Authorities Priorities for the Eighties. Edinburgh: HMSO, 1980 (SHAPE Report).

2. Scottish Home and Health Department. Scottish Health Authorities Review of Priorities for the Eighties and Nineties. Edinburgh: HMSO, 1988 (SHARPEN Report).

3. National Audit Office. Coronary Heart Disease. London: NAO, 1989.

4. King Edward's Hospital Fund for London. Blood Cholesterol Management in the Prevention of Coronary Heart Disease: Consensus Statement. London: King's Fund Centre, London, 1989.

5. Committee of Public Accounts. Coronary Heart Disease. London: HMSO, 1989.

6. World Health Organisation, Targets for health for all. Copenhagen: WHO, Regional Office for Europe, 1985.

7. Vemura K, Pisa Z. World Health Statistics Quarterly 1985; 38: 142-62.

8. Pisa Z, Vemura K. World Health Statistics Quarterly 1982; 35: 11-47.

9. Registrar General Scotland. Annual Report 1988. Edinburgh: HMSO, 1989.

10. Common Services Agency, Scottish Health Service. Scottish Health Statistics 1988. Edinburgh: CSA, 1988.

11. Common Services Agency, Scottish Health Service. Scottish Health Service Costs 1988. Edinburgh: CSA, 1988.

12. Office of Population Censuses and Surveys. Occupational Mortality—Decennial Supplement, 1986. London: OPCS, 1986.

13. Vemura K, Pisa Z. World Health Statistics Quarterly 1988; 41: 155-178.

14. National Forum for Coronary Heart Disease Prevention. Coronary Heart Disease Prevention—Action in the UK 1984-87. London: National Forum, 1988.

15. Kallio V, Cay E (eds.) Rehabilitation after Myocardial Infraction: the European Experience. World Health Organisation, 1985.

16. Ross R. The Pathogenesis of Arteriosclerosis—an update. New England Journal of Medicine 1986; 314: 488-500.

17. Davies M J. The Pathology of Ischaemic Heart Disease. In: Fox K M, ed. Ischaemic Heart Disease. Lancaster University Press, 1987: 33-68.

18. Fraser G E. Preventive Cardiology. Oxford University Press, 1986.

19. Arntzenius AC. Diet, Lipoproteins and the Progression of Coronary Atherosclerosis. The Leiden Intervention Trial. Drugs 1986; 31: suppl. 1: 61-5.

20. Blankerhorn DH et al. Beneficial Effects of Combined Colestipol Niacin Therapy on Coronary Atherosclerosis and Coronary Venous Bypass Grafts. Journal of the American Medical Association 1987; 257: 3233-40

21. Neaton J D, Tauller L H, Wentworth D, Borhani D. Total and cardiovascular mortality in relation to cigarette smoking, serum cholesterol concentrations and diastolic blood pressure among black and white males followed up for five years. American Heart Journal 1984; 108: 729.

22. Marmot M G and Mann J I. Epidemiology of Ischaemic Heart Disease. In: Fox K M, ed. Ischaemic Heart Disease. Lancaster University Press, 1987: 1-31.

23. Rose G, Shipley M. Plasma cholesterol concentration and deaths from coronary heart disease: 10 year results of the Whitehall study. British Medical Journal 1986; 293: 306-7.

24. Keys A. Seven Countries: Death and Coronary Heart Disease. Cambridge: Harvard University Press, 1980.

25. Frederickson D S, Lees R S. System for phenotyping hyperlipoproteinaemia. Circulation 1965; 31: 321.

26. Sherwin R et al. Serum Cholesterol Levels and Cancer Mortality in 361,662 Men Screened for the Multiple Risk Intervention Trial. Journal of the American Medical Association 1987; 275: 943-8.

27. Smith W C et al. Concomitance of Excess Coronary Deaths: Major Risk Factor and Lifestyle Findings from 10,359 Men and Women in the Scottish Heart Health Study. Scottish Medical Journal 1989; 34: 550-5.

28. Yusuf S, Wittes J, Friedman L. Overview of results of randomised clinical trials in heart disease. Journal of the American Medical Association 1988; 260: 2088-93, 2259-63.

29. Wells N. Coronary heart disease: the need for action. London: Office of Health Economics, 1987.

30. Meade T W et al. Haemostatic Function and Ischaemic Heart Disease: principal results of the Northwick Park Heart Study. Lancet 1986; 2: 533-7.

31. Health Education Authority. Health and Lifestyle: Report on a Survey of Knowledge, Attitudes and Behaviour. London: HEA, 1989.

32. Kannel W B, Gordon T. The Framingham Study—an epidemiological investigation of cardiovascular disease. National Institutes of Health, Washington, 1974 (74-599).

33. Sonne-Holm S, et al. Independent Effect of Weight Change and Attained Body Weight on Prevalence of Arterial Hypertension in Obese and Non-Obese Men. British Medical Journal 1989; 299: 767-70.

34. Slattery M L, Jacobs D R, Nichaman M Z. Leisure time physical activity and coronary heart disease death. Circulation 1989; 79; 304-11.

35. Sheppard R J. Exercise Physiology. Philadelphia: B C Becker Inc, 1987.

36. Sharkey B J. Physiology of Fitness. 2nd ed. Illionois. Human Kinetics Publishers, 1982.

37. American College of Sports Medicine. Guidelines for Exercise Testing and Prescription. Philadelphia: Lea and Febiger, 1986.

38. Hardman A E, Hudson A, Jones P R M, Norgan M G. Brisk walking and plasma high density lipoprotein cholesterol in previously sedentary women. British Medical Journal 1989; 299: 1204.

39. Jarret R J. Is there an ideal body weight? British Medical Journal 1986; 293: 493-5.

40. Steptoe A. Type A Coronary-Prone Behaviour. British Journal of Hospital Medicine, 1985; 33: 257-60.

41. Johnston D W, Cook D G, Shaper A G. Type A behaviour and ischaemic heart disease in middle aged British men. British Medical Journal 1987; 295: 86-9.

42. World Health Organisation. Prevention of Coronary Heart Disease. Geneva: WHO, 1982. (Technical report Series, No. 678)

43. Hutchison S J, Stamler J, Douglas A S. Changes in public awareness of coronary risk factors. Health Bulletin (Edinburgh) 1988; 46: 268.

44. Dayton S et al. A Controlled Trial of a Diet High in Unsaturated Fats in Preventing Complications of Arteriosclerosis. Circulation 1969; 39/40 (suppl 2): 1-63.

45. Turpeinen O et al. Dietary Prevention of Coronary Heart Disease: the Finnish Mental Hospitals Study. International Journal of Epidemiology 1979; 8: 99-118.

46. Lipid Research Clinics Programme: The Lipid Clinics Coronary Primary Prevention Trial Results: 1. Reduction in Incidence of Coronary Heart Disease. Journal of American Medical Association 1984; 251: 351-64.

47. Ibid. The Lipid Clinics Coronary Primary Prevention Trial Results: 2. The Relationship of Reduction in Incidence of Coronary Heart Disease to Cholesterol Lowering. Journal of American Medical Association 1984; 251: 365-74.

48. Frick M H et al. The Helsinki Heart Study. New England Journal of Medicine 1987; 317: 1237-45.

49. Rose G et al. A Randomised Controlled Trial of Anti-smoking Advice: 10 year results. Journal of Epidemiology and Community Health 1982; 36: 102-8.

50. Hjermann I et al. Effect of Diet and Smoking Intervention on Incidence of Coronary Heart Disease: report from Oslo Study Group of a Randomised Trial in Healthy Men. Lancet 1981; 2: 1303-10.

51. Multiple Risk Factor Intervention Trial—Risk Factor Changes and Mortality Results. Journal of the American Medical Association 1982; 248: 1465-77.

52. Cutler J A, Neaton J D, Hulley S B, Kuller L, Paul O, Stamler J. Coronary heart disease and all causes mortality in the Multiple Risk Factor Intervention Trial: subgroup findings and comparisons with other trials. Prev Med 1985; 14: 293.

53. Multiple Risk Factor Intervention Trial Research Group. Exercise Electrocardiogram and Coronary Heart Disease Mortality in the Multiple Risk Factor Intervention Trial. American Journal of Cardiology 1985; 55: 16-24.

54. WHO European Collaborative Group. European Collaborate Trial of Multi-factorial Prevention of Coronary Heart Disease. Final Report of the six year results. Lancet. 1986; 1: 896.

55. Wilhelmson L et al. The Multi-factorial Primary Prevention Trial in Goteborg, Sweden. European Heart Journal 1986; 7: 279-88.

56. Salonen J T et al. Decline in Mortality from Coronary Heart Disease in Finland from 1969 to 1979. British Medical Journal 1983; 286: 1857-60.

57. Salonen J T. Did the North Karelia project reduce coronary mortality? Lancet 1987; 2: 269.

58. Faculty of Community Medicine. Health for All by the Year 2000: Charter for Action. London: the Faculty, 1986.

59. World Health Organisation. Health For All: European Targets. Geneva: WHO, 1985.

60. Canadian Public Health Association. Ottawa Charter for Health Promotion. Geneva: WHO, 1986.

61. World Health Organisation. Constitution.

62. World Health Organisation. Health Promotion: Concept & Principles in Action. Geneva: WHO, 1986.

63. Tannahill A. What is Health Promotion? Health Education Journal: 1985; 44: 4.

64. Scottish Health Education Group. Be All You Can Be. Edinburgh: the Group.

65. World Health Organisation. Summary of Third Conference on Coronary Heart Disease. Geneva: WHO, 1984.

66. World Health Organisation. Lifestyles and their Impact on Health: Technical Discussion of 33 Session. Geneva: WHO, 1984.

67. Tones B K. Effectiveness and Efficiency in Health Education. A Review of Theory and Practice. Edinburgh: Scottish Health Education Unit, 1977.

68. Committee on Medical Aspects of Food Policy. Diet and Cardiovascular Disease. London: HMSO, 1984. (Reports on Health and Social Subjects No. 28.)

69. National Advisory Committee on Nutrition Education. Proposals for Nutritional Guidelines for Health Education in Britain. London: Health Education Council, 1983.

70. James W P T. Healthy Nutrition. Copenhagen: World Health Organisation, 1988. (European Series No. 24.)

71. Thomson M et al. Alcohol Consumption and Nutrient Intake in Middle-aged Scottish Men. American Journal of Clinical Nutrition 1988; 47: 139-45.

72. Smith W C et al. Urinary Electrolyte Excretions, Alcohol Consumption and Blood Pressure in the Scottish Heart Health Study. British Medical Journal 1988; 2: 329-30.

73. Heartbeat Wales. Personal communication. Cardiff: Health Promotion Authority for Wales.

74. Few W M. Prevalence of Cigarette Smoking in Dundee School Children in 1964 and 1984, Community Medicine 1985; 7: 283-8.

75. The Smoke Buster Club. Projected Management Report No. 8, 1987.

76. Schwartz J L. Smoking Cessation Methods. Washington: US Department of Health and Human Services, 1987.

77. Scottish Health Education Co-ordinating Committee. Health Education in the Prevention of Smoking-related Diseases. Edinburgh: Scottish Home and Health Department, 1983.

78. Health Education Council. Look After Yourself: Health Guide. London: the Council, 1986.

79. Scottish Health Education Co-ordinating Committee. Health Education and the Prevention of Alcohol Related Diseases. Edinburgh: Scottish Home and Health Department, 1985.

80. World Health Organisation. The World Health Organisation MONICA project (Monitoring trends and determinants in cardiovascular disease): a major international collaboration. Journal of Clinical Epidemiology 1988, 41: 105-14.

81. Vlietstra R, Kronmal R A, Oberman A, Frye R L, Killip T. Effect of cigarette smoking on survival of patients with angiographically documented coronary artery disease. JAMA 1986; 255: 1023-7.

82. Office of Population Censuses and Surveys. General Household Survey 1986. London: HMSO, 1987.

83. Marmot M G, Adelstein A M, Bulusu L. Lessons from the study of immigrant mortality. Lancet 1984; 1: 1455-7.

84. Broughton P M G et al. Quality of plasma cholesterol measurements in primary care. British Medical Journal 1989; 298: 297-8.

85. Inside Story. Cholesterol Testing. Which? September 1989: 412.

86. Swales J F D, Ramsay L E, Coope J R et al. Treating mild hypertension. British Medical Journal 1989; 298: 694.

87. Symposium on Alcohol. Proceedings of the Royal College of Physicians of Edinburgh 1989; 19: 267.

88. Fullard E et al. Facilitating Prevention in Primary Care. British Medical Journal 1984; 289: 1585-7.

89. Daines, Graham. Look After Yourself 1978-1986: Innovation and Outcomes. University of Nottingham, Department of Adult Education, 1986.

MEMBERSHIP OF WORKING GROUP

Dr W Keith Davidson, GP, Glasgow (Chairman).
Miss M Aitken, CANO, Greater Glasgow Health Board
(resigned December 1988).
Mrs H Anthony, CANO, Argyll and Clyde Health Board
(appointed February 1989).
Miss H Coubrough, Area Dietitian, Grampian Health Board.
Mr J C Currie, Unit General Manager, Monklands and Cumbernauld Unit,
Lanarkshire.
Dr H J Dargie, Consultant Cardiologist, Western Infirmary, Glasgow*
Mrs D Dey, Health Visitor, Livingston
(resigned May 1989).
Mr W S Fyfe, Chairman, Ayrshire and Arran Health Board.
Miss L Horn, Health Visitor, Edinburgh
(appointed May 1989).
Professor J G R Howie, University of Edinburgh
(resigned December 1988).
Dr I G Jones, CAMO, Fife Health Board.
Dr M McWhirter, Consultant in Public Health Medicine, Forth Valley
Health Board.
Mr J McWilliam, Chairman, Highland Health Board.
Mr S C Mitchell, Director, Scottish Health Education Group.
Mr D A Peters, General Manager, Borders Health Board.
Mr G Robertson, Area Health Education Officer, Lothian Health Board.
Dr W C Smith, Epidemiologist, University of Dundee†.

Assessors

Mr W F L Bigwood, HM Inspectorate, Scottish Education Department.
Mr L C Cunning, Scottish Home and Health Department
(until December 1988).
Miss H T McIntosh, Scottish Home and Health Department.
Dr A D McIntyre, Scottish Home and Health Department.
Mr R Milne, University of Glasgow
(from April 1989 to August 1989).
Mrs C Morgan, Scottish Home and Health Department
(from December 1988).

---

* Chairman of the Individual Strategy Sub-Group.
† Chairman of the Population Strategy Sub-Group.

Secretary

Mrs F M Cruickshanks, SHSAC Secretariat, Scottish Home and Health
Department.

C

SOURCES OF EVIDENCE CONSIDERED BY THE WORKING GROUP

(a) Individuals Presenting Evidence in Person

Miss P Birkett, Project Manager, Good Hearted Glasgow.

Professor S M Cobbe, Walton Professor of Cardiology, Royal Infirmary, Glasgow.

Dr L A G Davidson, Director, Good Hearted Glasgow.

Professor J V J A Durnin, Institute of Physiology, University of Glasgow.

Dr J S M Holms, GP, Alloway.

Dr D R Love, GP, Peebles.

Dr D V McQueen, Research Unit in Health and Behavioural Change, University of Edinburgh.

Dr M McWhirter, Co-Director, Be Better Hearted (Forth Valley).

Miss M Millar, Development Officer, Good Hearted Glasgow.

Mr R Milne, Department of Political Economy, University of Glasgow.

Mrs J Morgan, Facilitator, Be Better Hearted (Forth Valley).

Mr P Mouncey, Co-ordinator, Be Better Hearted (Forth Valley).

Dr A Tannahill, Department of Community Medicine, University of Glasgow.

Professor H Tunstall Pedoe, Cardiovascular Epidemiology Unit, Ninewells Hospital and Medical School, Dundee.

(b) Bodies Providing Written Evidence

COSLA.

Faculty of Occupational Medicine.

National Consultative Committee of Scientists—Clinical Psychology Sub-Committee.

National Dental Consultative Committee.

National Medical Consultative Committee.

National Nursing and Midwifery Consultative Committee.

National Paramedical Consultative Committee—Dietetics and Physiotherapy Sub-Committees.

National Pharmaceutical Consulative Committee.

A FRAMEWORK FOR A NATIONAL NUTRITION POLICY
BASED ON RECENT MAJOR REPORTS (1, 2 and 3)

(a) Total fat intake in the population as a mean should be reduced to 35% of total energy intake with 30% being the long term goal.

(b) Saturated fat intake in the population should be reduced to 15% of total energy intake with 10% being the long term goal.

(c) Polyunsaturated fatty acid intake in the population should be increased to 5% of total energy intake.

(d) The Polyunsaturated/Saturated ratio (P/S) should be increased to 0.32 with 0.45 being the long term goal.

(e) Intake of sugar should be not more than 12% of total energy intake.

(f) Fibre intake daily should be increased to 25 g and to 30 g in the long term.

(g) Salt intake should be decreased as it is considered to be needlessly high (1). The reduction should be by 1 g per day, and by 3 g per day in the long term.

(h) Alcohol intake should be reduced to 5% of total energy intake and to 4% or less in the long term. Reduction of the population mean intake will also reduce the numbers whose intake is excessive although such individuals may require targeted intervention.

(i) No change is recommended in the level of protein intake but some shift from animal to cereal and vegetable protein is recommended.

(j) Intake of carbohydrate should increase to compensate for the reduction in fat intake. This should be in the form of fruit, vegetables, bread and potatoes.

(k) Energy intake should be maintained because of the increased energy expenditure with the recommended increase in physical exercise.

(l) Mineral and vitamin intakes should be the UK recommended daily allowances.

NUTRITION POLICY RECOMMENDATIONS AND PRESENT NUTRITION IN SCOTLAND

| | Recommended Levels | | |
	Short-term	Long-term	Actual levels[61]
Percent energy			
Total fat	35%	30%	38.1%
Saturated fat	15%	10%	16.3%
Polyunsaturated fat	5%	5%	4.6%
Sugar	12%	12%	—
Alcohol	5%	4%	6.7%
Protein	11%	11%	13.6%
Carbohydrate	49%	55%	41.4%
P/S ratio	0.32	0.45	0.30
Fibre g/day	25.00	30.00	19.80
Salt decrease g/day	1.00	3.00	11.60[62]

Source:

ACTION ON RISK FACTORS

Risk factor	Criterion for intervention	Target	Action by		
			Primary care assessment staff	GP	Others
High blood cholesterol	5.2–6.5 mmol	5.2	Advice on healthy eating/weight reduction at initial assessment session	—	—
	6.5–10.0 mmol	5.2	As above, followed by further session to monitor progress/re-inforce advice. If appropriate, refer to GP	Further counselling; refer to lipid clinic if necessary	Specialist treatment including dietitian
	10.0 mmol	5.2	Refer to GP	Refer to lipid clinic	Specialist treatment including dietitian
Smoking	<20 cigarettes per day	Stop or reduce consumption	Counselling at initial assessment session	—	—
	20 cigarettes or more per day	Stop or reduce consumption	As above, followed, as appropriate, by further counselling session. Attendance at smoking group and referral to GP	Further counselling. Consideration of acupuncture, hypnotherapy or nicotine chewing gum	—
High blood pressure	Diastolic BP 95–109 mmHg	Diastolic BP <95 mmHg	Lifestyle advice at initial assessment session, further review	—	—
	Diastolic BP ≥110 mmHg	Diastolic BP <95 mmHg	Refer to GP	Counselling: drugs if appropriate	—
Exercise	Below target	Pulse at resting rate + (220 − age) × 60% for 20–30 mins 3 times per week	Advice and encouragement	Medical examination prior to exercise if appropriate	—
Obesity	Weight 20% or more above normal for height/sex	Normal weight for height/sex	Dietary, etc counselling, support groups. Refer extreme cases to dietitian	—	Counselling. Advice and training to other staff by dietitian

Table 1

TRENDS IN AGE SPECIFIC CORONARY HEART DISEASE MORTALITY RATES IN SCOTTISH MEN FROM 1968

(Rates per 100,000)

Year	Age in years					
	40–	45–	50–	55–	60–	65–
1968	115	257	416	662	1,064	1,646
1969	117	235	434	729	1,088	1,635
1970	114	245	444	705	1,110	1,659
1971	119	289	437	705	1,075	1,659
1972	147	241	483	750	1,177	1,744
1973	131	264	482	794	1,138	1,717
1974	130	273	453	781	1,113	1,676
1975	120	267	426	730	1,074	1,676
1976	108	239	438	716	1,148	1,664
1977	108	229	460	692	1,130	1,600
1978	107	246	461	720	1,136	1,729
1979	111	357	472	717	1,172	1,653
1980	105	236	438	722	1,088	1,525
1981	97	262	450	679	1,070	1,523
1982	88	225	390	683	1,069	1,553
1983	94	231	420	705	1,098	1,553
1984	84	213	382	681	990	1,635
1985	93	190	349	613	1,056	1,552
1986	83	195	366	662	1,006	1,505
1987	81	176	364	582	1,034	1,458
1988	72	173	325	582	952	1,504

Source: World Health Organisation.

Table 2

PHYSICAL ACTIVITY AT WORK AND LEISURE

Percentage of males and females aged 40–59 who are active at work (self-reported) or take part in vigorous activity (at least three times per week, lasting 20 minutes, during which participants are short of breath and perspire)

| | Active | | Vigorous activity | |
	At work %	At leisure %	At work %	At leisure %
Male	42	23	18	14
Female	47	19	14	10

Source: Scottish Heart Health Study.

Table 3

PREVALENCE OF MAJOR RISK FACTORS* IN THE SCOTTISH POPULATION

	Male	Female
Percentage with		
No risk factors	32	32
1 risk factor	46	45
2 risk factor	20	21
3 risk factor	2	2

* Major risk factors were defined as:—
    Blood cholesterol of 6.5 or over.
    Smoking.
    Diastolic blood pressure of 100 or over.

Source: Scottish Heart Health Study.

Table 4

HEALTH PROMOTION INITIATIVES BY HEALTH BOARDS, SEPTEMBER 1989

A.

Type of programme	In progress	Planned, not yet implemented	Plans in progress	No current plans	All
CHD	4*	1	5	5	15
Nutrition	8	2	4	1	15
Smoking	12	1	1	1	15

* 2 implemented in full, 2 in part.

B. Boards with CHD Programmes in Progress or Planned

Type of programme	In progress	Planned, not yet implemented	Plans in progress	No current plans	All
Nutrition	5	2	3	—	10
Smoking	8	1	1	—	10

C. Boards with No Current Plans for CHD Programmes

Type of programme	In progress	Plans in progress	No current plans	All
Nutrition	3	1	1	5
Smoking	4	—	1	5

FIGURE 1:

DEATHS BY CAUSE, BY SEX AND AGE GROUP, OVER 35, SCOTLAND 1988

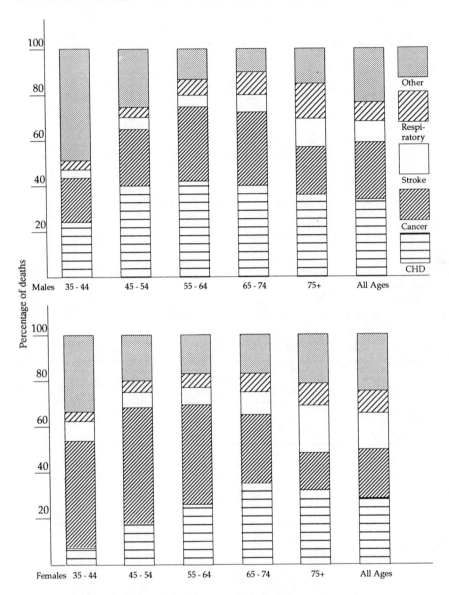

Source: Registrar General Scotland, Annual Report 1988.

SOCIAL CLASS DIFFERENCES IN CORONARY HEART DISEASE MORTALITY
FOR MEN AGED 15–64 YEARS (UK)

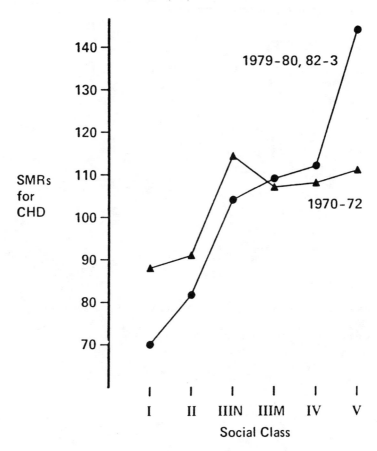

Source: OPCS[12].

FIGURE 3:

TRENDS IN CORONARY HEART DISEASE MORTALITY RATES FOR WOMEN AGED 40–69 YEARS, 1968–86
Age-adjusted rates per 100,000 for certain countries

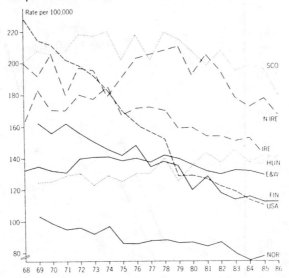

TRENDS IN CORONARY HEART DISEASE MORTALITY RATES FOR MEN AGED 40–69 YEARS, 1968–86
Age-adjusted rates per 100,000 for certain countries

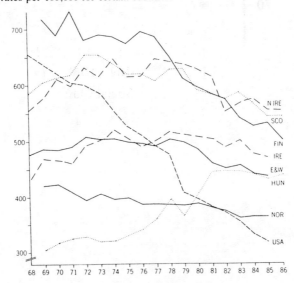

Source: Cardiovascular Epidemiology Unit, Dundee[14].

76

FIGURE 4:

DEATH RATES FROM CORONARY HEART DISEASE, BY AGE AND SEX,
SCOTLAND, 1987

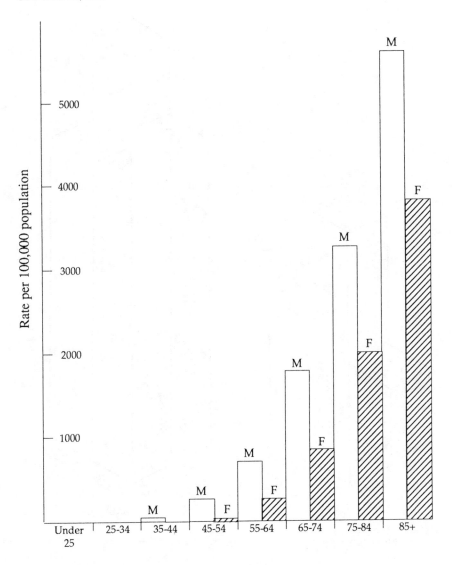

Source: Scottish Health Statistics 1988.

FIGURE 5:
INTERACTION OF RISK FACTORS

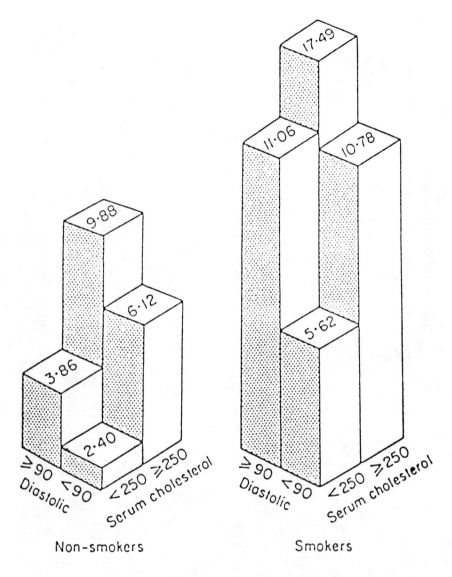

Source: Multiple Risk Factor Intervention trial.

Printed by HMSO, Edinburgh Press
Dd 0287412 C50 3/90 (278038)